Success Stories

I subsequently have dropped in weight from 188 pounds to 170 pounds in six weeks. I get compliments multiple times a day, and am in better shape and have a more muscular physique than my several nephews that are in their early twenties. I have tremendous energy during the day, I am never hungry, and I sleep like a stress-free rock!

Tom Lacey, M.D.
Board Certified, Internal Medicine

Yes, it took me ten months and some willpower and resolve to get down to my current weight of 245 pounds, but that is down 65 pounds from the day I went to buy the "fat clothes" and I am not finished yet! I am thankful each day that I had a professional like Dr. Hashim, who took an interest in sharing his knowledge with a patient and guiding me on the right path to a better me.

Frank McDowell, III

Now twelve weeks later, I've already lost 49 pounds without missing a meal or ever feeling hungry. Taking ninety percent of your advice with ten percent of my tweaking to accommodate my personal tastes, allowed me to buy into the philosophy. I'm well on my way to the 'new, lighter' me.

Gary Blumberg

With his help, by following his program, I have lost 63 pounds. I feel like a new person! THANK YOU DR. HASHIM!!!

Chad Waltz

I have lost over 55 pounds and I feel great, and look great. And as you know, there are no more shots for me. If folks will try your program Doc, it will change their lives forever. I am living proof.

Paul Hloska

HEALTHY FOR LIFE NOW

For Spencer, Parker and Sophia…
you are the true inspiration for my life.

Healthy For Life Now

"If you let life get in the way of your health,
your health will get in the way of your life."™

By Mark N. Hashim, M.D.
Board Certified, American Board of Anesthesiologists

President,
CFN Concepts, LLC
Healthy For Life Now, LLC
Cosmetic Fitness and Nutrition, LLC

Edited by Christine Robson, CRNA, ARNP

ISBN 13: 978-0-9831913-0-8

Contact information:

www.CosmeticFitnessandNutrition.com
www.MarkHashimMD.com
www.CFNconcepts.com

CONTENTS

Acknowledgments

First and foremost I must thank my beautiful wife, Christine. Since our marriage in 1997, she has turned my world into something I only dreamt about. She has been the solid rock that has supported me no matter what; she is not only an outstanding wife, more importantly she is the most amazing mother. She has given birth to three of the most loving, caring and gifted children anyone could ask for. I love them all so much and they mean the world to me. They are truly my inspiration. I take care of myself so that I can be around to watch and enjoy them grow.

Spencer, Parker and Sophia, I love you with all my heart and soul. May your days be bright and cheerful. May you face adversity with a smile. May you achieve all that you hope for in life and more. But most of all, may you enjoy each other's company as much as I enjoy yours. Hug, kiss, nose kiss, butterfly kiss, head butt to boot, I love you, toot, toot, rat (princess).

It's so easy cavemen did it...
and YOU can too!

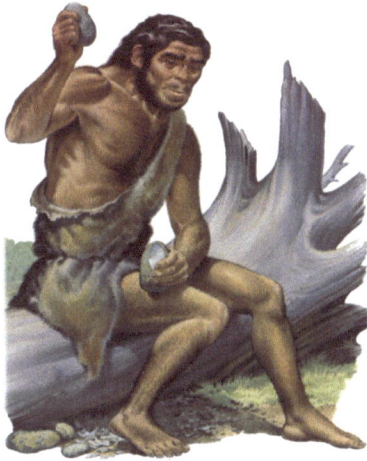

Introduction

"If you let life get in the way of your health, your health will get in the way of your life."™

I believe the above statement summarizes why eating healthy and exercising is so vital to your body. Remember: you control what you do to your body and what you place in your body.

So here's the deal. You're over 30 years old, you are not feeling great and you just went to the doctor. You used to be a relatively fit person, maybe a cheerleader or football player, but you have let yourself go. You probably have a large gut or thighs and you get short of breath when you go upstairs or play with your children. Maybe you are a female who wants some curves back or maybe you are a guy who wants to be fitter and trimmer. You look in the mirror and you want to scream because you want to change – **big time** – but no one tells you how.

Your doctor checks you out, offers a couple prescription medications that cost hundreds of dollars and says to come back in a couple of months. His parting words are, "Your blood pressure is high, you've got high cholesterol, you might become diabetic and you need to lose weight." He doesn't explain how to lose the weight or why losing it can reverse most of the medical problems you are having.

If this sounds familiar, then **you need ME**. You need me because I am a Medical Doctor who is in excellent physical shape. I have run marathons and triathlons, won several power lifting competitions and recovered from left arm and chest paralysis to WIN a body building competition. I have been involved in physical fitness for over 35 years and I know how to lose the weight and keep it off. I know how to get **your** body running like a lean, mean fighting machine... if you want. Or you can take the pills and the vitamin shots, gain more weight and continue to feel miserable until you die a premature death, leaving your kids and loved ones to bury you.

So what's it going to be? Would you rather live a healthy life or wait for the heart attack, the stroke, the arthritis that eats up your joints or the kidney failure that will be your wake-up call?

The problem is, once you develop those problems, there is no turning back. I know because I have seen thousands of elderly patients in my Pain Management practice and almost every single one says, "Doc, I wish I took better care of myself when I was younger." Or, like famed Yankee Mickey Mantle once said, "**If I'd known I was gonna live this long, I would have taken better care of myself.**"
YOU CAN NOT TURN THE CLOCK BACK. But you can help prevent problems if you act now. Two things: you must

eat right and you must exercise. If you do not, be prepared to get sick and die before you have the chance to enjoy a full life.

So why come to me? I see thousands of patients who do not take care of themselves and I see what neglect leads to. I choose to lead by example, which means exercising and eating correctly myself. How can an overweight and out of shape doctor be taken seriously by patients when he says, "You need to lose weight, eat right and exercise"?

I am living proof and so are those who follow my plan. I have coached numerous clients into a successful, healthy lifestyle change. One of my clients is Paul, a patient of mine for many years. He was about 80 pounds overweight, had a huge gut and could barely walk up a flight of stairs without huffing or puffing. He could not sleep and his gut affected numerous aspects of his life – you get the picture. One day in my office, I said to Paul, "What the heck are you doing? You're a time bomb waiting to explode and at this rate, you're **not** going to make it to fifty. I guarantee it." Paul asked, "What do I do, Doc?" My response? "Just do what I tell you to do." That is when I started him on my wholesome foods and fitness program. He listened and did exactly what I said with no ifs ands or buts.

Paul is now fifty pounds lighter, never gets short of breath, looks like a million bucks and his friends say he looks five years younger. He tells me he feels like he is thirty and full of life. His cholesterol and blood pressure are perfect and he works out like a 20 year old. How do I know that? I know because he is my patient and my workout partner. He is living proof that my simple, no-bull program works **and it will work for you.**

Wake up and smell the coffee. Every day you waste is another day you are staring death in the eyes.

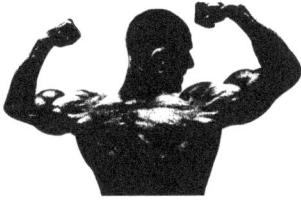

1

Why Can't My Health Care Provider Do This for Me?

I will tell you a funny story. I was working out in my home gym and I saw my neighbor running down the street. He is an extremely intelligent physician, 52 years old and about twenty pounds overweight. I was thrilled to see him running because he had commented to me how he wanted to get into shape. I invited him into my gym. After talking about his goals to lose weight, I asked about how and what he eats. I could not believe my ears – he had no idea how to eat correctly and he was making all of the same mistakes the average Joe makes. In fact, my auto body repair man used to follow the same wrong food choices and he had a big gut before he met me and started to change. It is amazing how unfit the average health care provider is, especially since they should know better. An overweight health care provider cannot instruct you on weight loss because if he knew what he was doing, he would not be overweight.

My point is, most health care providers do not know fitness and do not know proper nutrition – that is why they cannot help you. But I can help. I know how the body works and I can coach you on how to fuel the machine and get the results you desire, just like I have done with Paul

and numerous other patients.   As Paul always tells me,
"Doc, you're the real deal."

Most health care providers learn to treat your medical
problems. I prevent problems. My plan is very simple, so
let's work together.

Follow my plan and you can turn yourself around.

In fact, in a year you will be amazed at the results if you
follow the plan. I know the road and how to drive down it
and you need to sit in the car and enjoy the road.

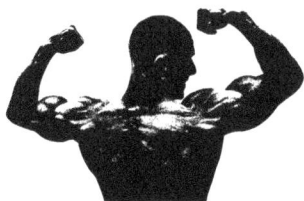

2

Speaking of Rides, How Does the Body Machine Work?

Everyone has a truck, car or some kind of gas powered machine with thousands of moving parts. Everyone has a body with thousands of moving parts. When you go to the gas station, what would happen if you accidentally put water in the gas tank or filled it with diesel instead of unleaded? The machine wouldn't work, right? What if you put low octane in your precious vehicle? Well it works, but it knocks and pings and is not as efficient as it could be. What if you never changed the oil? Wouldn't the sludge build up and break the engine? Of course it would. So, simple as it sounds, putting the wrong food in your body is just like putting the wrong fuel in your vehicle. The grade of fuel determines how well the machine works. Neglect the oil changes and the machine breaks.

The Tale of Two Cars

Let's look at two similar, brand new cars. One is treated extremely well by its owner. He uses the correct fuel, changes the oil as directed by the owner's manual, gets regular check-ups and changes wearing parts over time. He keeps the vehicle covered when not in use and washes and waxes the outside once a week. He is meticulous about the cabin and uses products to protect the interior from everyday wear and tear. You can bet that this vehicle will last the owner a very long time and become a classic.

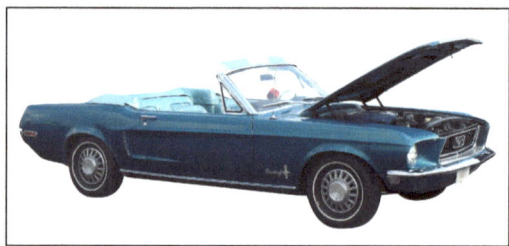

The other car is not so lucky. The owner uses inexpensive gasoline, forgets to change the oil and does not check or replace fluids. He entirely ignores the owner's manual. He never washes the exterior, leaves his trash on the floor and parks under pine trees. The second vehicle runs and looks like crap and it will not last very long. Every time it is driven, it runs the risk of falling apart or breaking down and never running again. Which of these would you rather own?

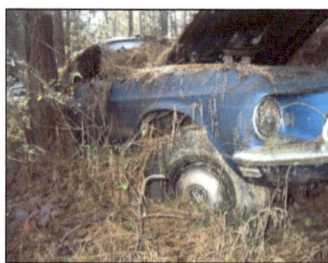

If you are not automotive minded, let's consider a pair of twins. One stays active and exercises every day regardless of the circumstances. He eats like a caveman (there's that caveman reference you have been waiting for), only drinks water, avoids snacks, protects his skin from the sun, visits his doctor regularly and is the "picture of health." The other twin watches television all day and gets up only so he can eat and go to the restroom. His food choices consist of fast food meals, potato chips and two liters of soda a day. When he goes outside, he never protects his skin from the sun and he rarely visits the doctor. Any time he exerts himself, he runs the risk of collapsing from a heart attack.

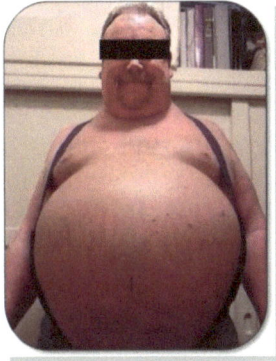

Which body would <u>you</u> rather have? The one in the above photo or the 47-year-old author of this book?

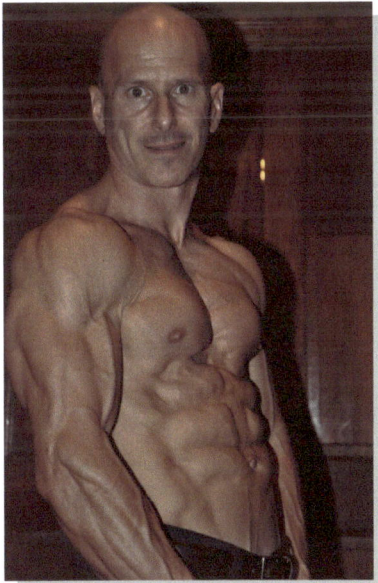

I hope you realize that the first car I described and the first twin share plenty. They are both lean, mean fighting machines. They look and feel great. Everyone stares at them and wonders how they look so good. Over time, the poorly kept vehicle becomes a piece of rusty, nonfunctional junk and the second twin becomes an overweight person with a lot of medical problems. The car gets mashed flat at the junkyard. The man dies at the age of forty from a sudden heart attack or suffers a stroke and cannot use one side of his body. Maybe he develops diabetes and loses his eyesight, or his kidneys fail and he has to sleep in a recliner so he will not get too short of breath.

There is hope for the second vehicle. A smart mechanic and auto body repair man could buy the piece of junk 1969 Mustang and renovate it. They set up a plan, execute that plan and work every day, carefully following the plan, replacing parts and rebuilding the car. Two years later, they will have a very valuable lean, mean fighting machine.

There is hope for the second twin, too. He reads this manual written by me and uses it exactly as it is intended to be used. Every day he makes the changes that are recommended. Every day he writes his goal down on a mirror and stares at it. The only fluids he drinks other than water are the occasional coffee or tea. He decreases his daily calories, stops the snacks and fast food and begins to eat like the first twin. He starts to walk further every day and before long, he is walking one mile, then two, then three. He notices that he is no longer short of breath. His children are delighted that dad gets to play with them. He sleeps better. His joints no longer ache; he looks thinner in the mirror. Suddenly, it is no longer painful when he squats down and his low back does not hurt when he walks. Chronic aches and pains begin to disappear. He feels better inside and out and remembers he felt the same way when he was younger. His friends begin to take notice and every time someone says, "Hey, you're looking good, man!", he feels better about himself. After two years, just like the renovated vehicle, he too looks and feels like a million bucks.

So, you don't think you can do this? You can't be renovated? Yes you can and you will **if** you do what I say. One key to this program is to make a mental vision of what you want to look and feel like. Remember how great you felt in your earlier years? You could run around and play all day (and sometimes all night) – never got tired, felt full of energy and slept soundly. You can and will regain those feelings if you follow my plan and make small steps on a daily basis. There is no safer weight loss program out there. So what are you waiting for? The time is now.

Statistics from the American Heart Association
(American Heart Association, 2010)

- About 600,000 people in the U.S. per year die from heart disease

- Forty percent of people age 40 - 59 have cardiovascular disease (leads to heart attack, stroke and death)

- 355,000 people per year age 45 - 64 have a heart attack

- 39% of people age 45-54 have high blood pressure, the silent killer

- The average American consumes 150 calories a day from sodas, 100 from alcohol and 77 from fruit juices and fruit drinks. That is 119,355 calories a year which equals 29 pounds of fat. (By drinking water, you could lose close to 30 pounds in one year, not to mention the money you would save)

- Two out of every three American adults and one out of every three children are obese

"It's difficult to avoid obesity in a toxic food environment," says Kelly Brownell (2010), a professor at Yale University, "because people who are exposed to [our food environment] get sick. They develop chronic diseases like diabetes and obesity in record numbers." (p. 1, 3)

Excess pounds raise the risk of diabetes, heart disease, stroke, cancer, gallbladder disease, arthritis and more. Once people gain weight, the odds of losing it and keeping it off are slim. Recent estimates are that the next generation will be the first to live fewer years than their parents. (Brownell, 2010)

People who have lost weight burn fewer calories than those who have not, so they have to continue taking in fewer calories to keep the weight off. This explains why rewarding yourself with cheat meals will lead to weight gain. Once you have reached your goal, you will have to continue consuming those lower daily calories and that means changing your environment conditions. Eat right and exercise more and you will begin to move in the right direction. (Brownell, 2010)

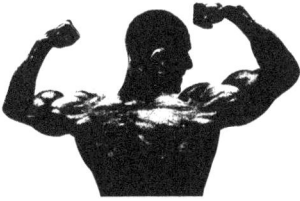

3

All Calories are Not Created Equal

Calorie is the word we use to describe a unit of energy for food items. There are good energy sources and there are bad energy sources. When you get gas for your car, the energy is measured by octane. We all know the high octane is a better choice for your vehicle. In the food world, natural foods that come from the earth are better energy sources than processed foods. Foods from the earth are high octane fuels; processed foods are low octane fuels. Remember this when you are shopping the grocery store aisles: if cavemen could eat the food you see, it is good for you. If factories have created the food, it is not so beneficial.

For example, look at your average "healthy" granola bar. If it is full of ingredients you cannot understand, do you think your body understands what to do with it? Did cavemen have high maltose corn syrup? I don't think so. That would be like putting gasoline with small amounts of dirt in your car – over time, it will destroy your engine. Good energy comes from nature and not so good energy comes from factories. I cannot emphasize this enough:

There is no way that our bodies were designed to consume man-made chemicals intended to keep foods from spoiling.

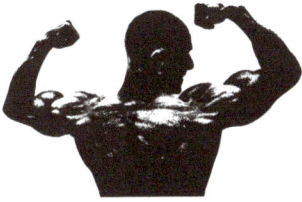

4

America Runs on Junkin'

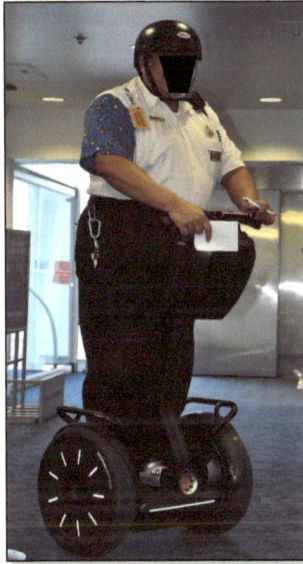

USA Airport Security

Chemicals poison every cell in your body and lead to multiple diseases like cancer, heart disease, diabetes and other problems. So why would you eat foods that cause those problems? Did you know that an artificial coloring called cochineal is found in candy, ice cream, yogurt, and beverages? Did you know that cochineal comes from the dried and crushed bodies of insects? Yummy – can't wait to eat that.

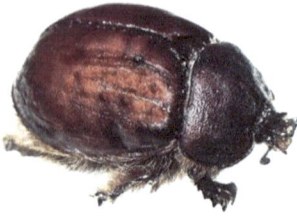

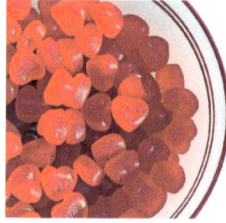

Nearly every food we consume from factories has high fructose corn syrup, which is largely responsible for type 2 diabetes, obesity, tooth decay and, when combined with a patient suffering from high triglycerides, can lead to potential heart disease. (Jacobson, 2008) Why would you do that to yourself? Are you aware that those potato chips, cereal packages and cooking oils contain BHA (butylated hydroxyanisole), which, according to our government's National Toxicology Program, is "reasonably anticipated to be a human carcinogen," which means it causes cancer? (Jacobson, 2008)

Still want that chip?

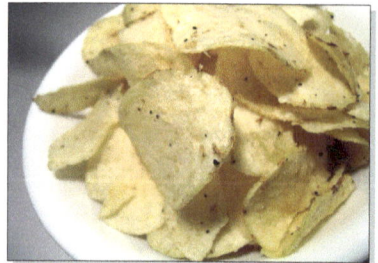

Because of our everyday conveniences, we are constantly eating more food than we need. If you eat more calories than you burn during the course of the day, your body stores that excess energy as fat. This is because caveman had no idea where his next meal would come from, so he stored fat for energy. Today, we eat constantly and we usually eat high calorie foods and drinks. If you always eat more than you need, then you get fatter and fatter. If you take in fewer calories than your body needs, then you shrink the fat cells and lose weight – and get leaner and leaner. Let me guide you on the good, the bad and the ugly. That is what I am trained to do.

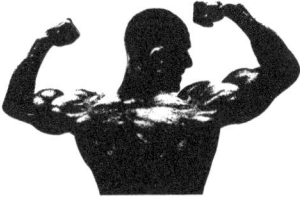

5

How Many Calories Do I Really Need a Day?

The formula for this is simple. Take your ideal body weight and multiply by ten. This is your daily requirement of calories. If you go over this, you gain weight. If you stay under this, you lose weight. If your ideal body weight is 160 pounds, then you only need 1600 calories a day. There are internet sites that will calculate your ideal body weight or you can use the formula below. To convert pounds to kilograms (kg), take the pounds and divide by 2.2.

To calculate your ideal body weight:

Estimate Ideal body weight in kilograms (kg) then convert to pounds

Males: IBW = 50 kg + 2.3 kg for each inch over 5 feet
(ex. 5'11" is 50kg + 2.3 (11) = 75.3kg x 2.2 = 166 pounds IBW)

Females: IBW = 45.5 kg + 2.3 kg for each inch over 5 feet
(ex. 5'4" is 45.5 kg + 2.3 (4) = 54.7kg x 2.2 = 120 pounds IBW)

Fill in the blank:

Males:
50 kg + 2.3 x (# of inches over 5 ft) = _____ kg x 2.2
= _____ pounds.

Females:
45.5kg + 2.3 x (# of inches over 5 ft) = ____kg x 2.2
= _____ pounds.

Let me introduce you to the Good, the Bad and the Ugly (Calories!)

Good calories are derived from foods that come from the earth and are not of a processed nature. The bad and the ugly are what we get from fast food chains and highly processed foods found in the aisles at the grocery store. Don't forget that crushed beetles are found in candy, beverages and ice cream. Cancer causing agents, according to the government, are found in cooking oils, chips and other processed foods. High fructose corn syrup ruins your teeth and can lead to type 2 diabetes. (Jacobson, 2008)

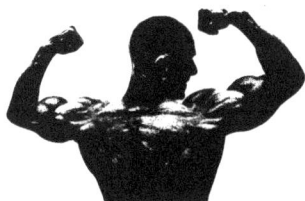

6

How Narcotics and Processed Foods are the Same

I am a Pain Management physician. I see thousands of patients who unfortunately must take narcotics. I am not in favor of this, but there are some strong comparisons between narcotics and poor diets that feature mainly processed foods. Both cause the person to want and desire the product (either the drug or the food), making them very addictive. Getting off of both is extremely difficult for some and takes persistence. So just like coming off of a drug, coming off of processed foods may cause you to feel uneasy and uncomfortable at first. But just like the drug addict, once you are off the drug or processed foods, you will start feeling like you used to feel – full of life and vigor.

Why don't starvation diets work?

My patients tell me that they don't understand why they can't lose weight. They all share very common misunderstandings about how the body works, therefore their approach does not work. The person typically skips breakfast, drinks juices or sodas during the day and eats a large dinner before bed. The problem is that the body is designed to receive food upon awakening and then food every two or three hours. If you skip breakfast, your body will break down protein for energy, so you lose muscle and the building blocks for your inside organs.

Most people make the big mistake of assuming that if you do not eat your body will break down fat. That is not going to happen. The <u>last</u> thing your body breaks down for energy is fat. So yes, you may lose the weight, but you lose it in the form of muscle. Over time, you will become "skinny fat," which translates to no tone, flabby skin, not very good-looking and feeling horrible.

If, instead, you eat upon awakening and then eat my healthy suggestions as outlined on the following pages, you will retain your building blocks and look more toned. If you start to exercise, you will destroy fat in a slow, methodical way, which means you will be able to maintain a healthy weight and probably reverse numerous medical problems.

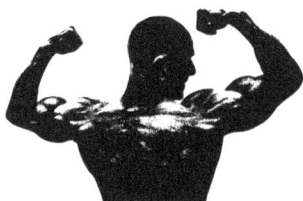

7

Make These Easy Food Choices Like the Cavemen Did

My food recommendations are simple and straight forward. I have outlined how to walk the walk. It may appear very strict and you may need to wean yourself off the bad foods that you consume then switch to these food choices over a period of five to ten days.

You will not be able to stick to these wholesome foods all the time, but if you can stick to them 50 – 75% of the time and make relatively healthy choices the rest of the time, you will make huge changes within a year and that is your goal. These are not novel ideas, just a new approach to the challenges of eating in an "on-the-go life." If you plan ahead and have healthy food nearby, you will not fail. Start your day correctly; do not poison your body. You wouldn't put the wrong fuel in your car so let me help you with the correct fuel for you.

Begin the day with ½ cup of oatmeal topped with ½ teaspoon of cinnamon (150 calories). You can prepare this the night before by placing the oatmeal (regular, not instant) and ½ teaspoon cinnamon in a container and barely covering it with water. Cover and store it in your refrigerator overnight. It is ready to eat in the morning with no need for additional cooking. Add an apple or a banana (roughly 100 calories) for a total of 250 healthy, unprocessed calories. You have used only 15% of your daily calories, so you could eat five more meals of 250 calories throughout the day.

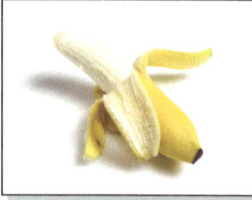

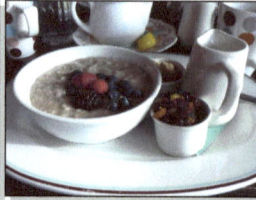

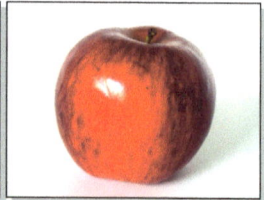

If instead you stopped at your favorite doughnut or coffee chain and ordered a bagel with cream cheese (450 calories) and a medium mocha coffee (350 calories), you would consume over 800 calories – more than half of your daily requirement if you weigh 160 pounds! Good luck staying under 1600 calories if you started your day this way.

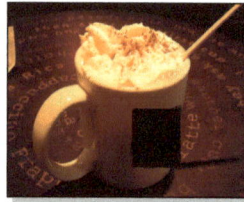

DO NOT SKIP BREAKFAST
Starving yourself does not lead to healthy weight loss.

Make sure you have all the water you need for the day with you.　Water should be your fluid source.　Man survived for thousands of years with water as his fluid source.　I usually fill three 64 ounce containers with filtered tap water and place in the refrigerator so they are ready to go in the morning.　Avoid sodas, diet drinks and fruit juices. These can fill you with empty carbohydrate calories that turn to fat.　**Do not drink sodas.**　One 12 ounce can of soda has about 150 calories.　If you drink three sodas a day you have consumed 450 calories and that is over 25% of your total caloric need (assuming an ideal body weight of 160 pounds).　This leads to tremendous weight gains as stored fat. It also translates to 164,250 calories a year! If you take 164,250 calories and divide by 9 calories/gram of fat that is 18.25 kilograms, which equals forty pounds of fat!

THREE SODAS EVERY DAY EQUALS NINETY POUNDS OF SUGAR A YEAR!

This equals FORTY POUNDS of FAT per YEAR!

If you replace the soda with water, it is zero calories and no fat.

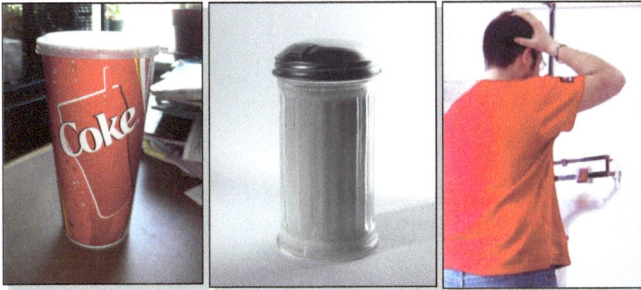

Conquering Your Snack Attack

Try to avoid all snacks between meals. If you really need some energy, try a protein shake like Beverly International's Ultimate Muscle Protein (UMP) that delivers 130 calories, eighty of which come from protein.

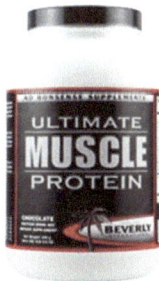

Another option is to try one of the following choices: 1/4 cup of almonds, sunflower seeds, a small salad, a piece of fruit, low fat cheese, low fat cottage cheese or some vegetables.

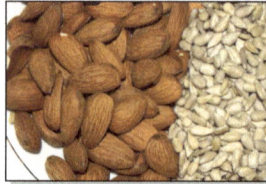

Remember to only eat a small amount and the hunger will disappear in twenty minutes. Also remember to drink water with your snack as it will help you feel fuller.

Two hours after breakfast, eat your next meal. You could have a large salad with lettuce, cucumbers, tomatoes, carrots or virtually any leafy green. Avoid croutons and fat-laden dressings. Use three to six ounces of lean meat or garbanzo beans, black beans or a half cup of any kind of bean. If salad is not an option, have steamed or roasted vegetables (without butter) with three to six ounces of lean meat and a bowl of fruit. If you are going to a restaurant, go for salads. Try to avoid wraps, burgers and fries. Alternatively, Taco Bell® has the option of ordering "Fresco style" which replaces fat-laden sauces and cheese with chopped tomatoes, onions and cilantro. Chick-Fil-A® has a grilled chicken sandwich with only 3.5 grams of fat. If you do order a sandwich, throw away the bread or at least the top half of the bun. A large fast food burger, large fries and a 24-ounce soda totals 1,350 calories – almost three-quarters of your daily calorie allotment in one meal! Be VERY careful of salad dressings at fast food restaurants. Most of them contain 200-300 calories per serving and will destroy the good intention of ordering a salad. If you eat a very large salad with half a skinless chicken breast and no dressing or only balsamic vinegar, your intake would be 200 calories at most. Selecting from my whole food recommendations will give you one-sixth of your daily caloric needs in a very healthy meal. Between meals, drink plenty of water.

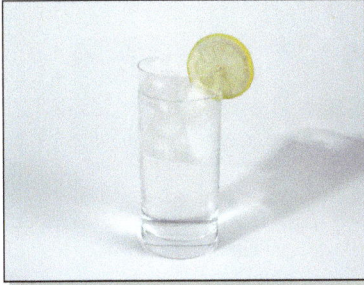

Three hours after your last meal, eat another meal using similar foods to the above which is again, 175 to 250 calories. You should consume multiple small meals every two to three hours.

Choose **ONE** from each category:

Protein: six egg whites or 4 - 6 oz. grilled skinless chicken breast, pork tenderloin, grilled top sirloin, 93% ground beef burger, grilled fish like tilapia, tuna or salmon

Carbohydrate: half of a medium sized sweet potato, two ounces whole grain pasta, ½ cup cooked brown rice or any type of fruit

Fiber: twelve ounces leafy greens or six ounces steamed broccoli, cauliflower, snap peas or your favorite vegetables (steamed, grilled, or roasted)

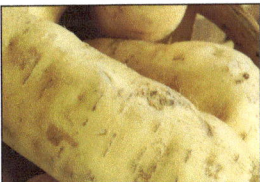

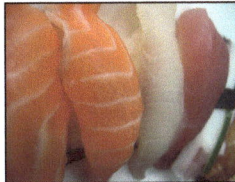

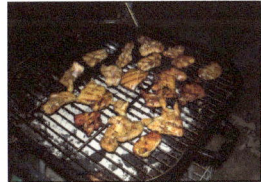

Fresh fish with brown rice and snapped peas makes a very healthy choice. Always do the math. You can have five meals a day like this one:

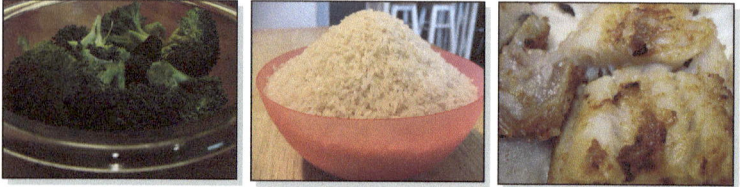

... **OR**... only <u>**ONE**</u> meal like this! So... what's it going to be?

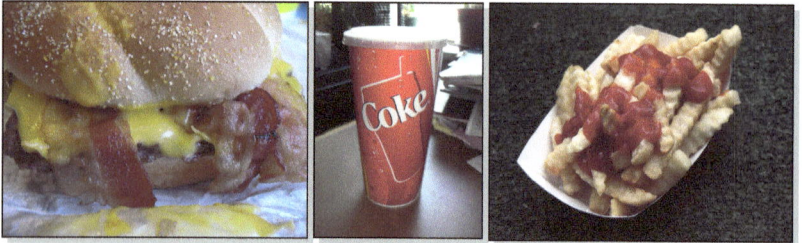

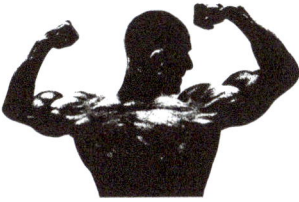

8

So Where Do All My Calories Go?

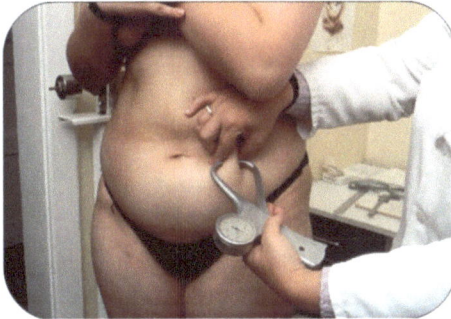

You got it – straight to fat.

> **Remember**: Multiple meals give your body the constant correct fuel it needs.

MY WAY: Each meal is about 175 – 250 calories, so you eat four to six small meals a day and only consume 1,000 – 1,500 calories.

WRONG WAY: Morning bagel with cream cheese and a mocha coffee for breakfast (800 calories), large fast food burger, large fries and a 24-ounce soda for lunch (1350 calories), four slices of pizza with the works and a 24-ounce soda for dinner (1612 calories). Throw in three more 12-ounce sodas throughout the day (450 calories) and you have taken in 4,212 calories – more than <u>double</u> what you need! By my calculations, those extra calories will make 0.6 pounds of fat <u>a day.</u>   Keep that up and you will gain <u>eighteen pounds in one month</u>.

Let's say you are a busy lady and this is your diet: cinnamon raisin bagel (440 calories) with a Venti Latté (340 calories), followed by a lunch that includes a chicken burrito supreme (444 calories) with a sweet iced tea (anywhere from 220 to 480 calories) and for dinner, ¼ fried chicken (414 calories), oven-heated steak fries (202 calories) with ketchup (45 calories), a glass of wine (148 calories) and finish with a peach cobbler (420 calories). Your total consumed for the day is between 2,673 and 2,933 calories.

If you are 5'3", you should weigh about 115 pounds and only consume 1,150 calories a day.   If your diet is like the above, you have taken in 1,730 calories more than your daily need... so you have gained 0.5 pounds of fat in ONE day. Keep that up and you'll gain 15.5 pounds per month. If you follow my advice and stay at ten calories per pound of ideal body weight per day, you would start to lose 2.2 pounds a month – which is 26 pounds a year! **THAT IS JUST BY CHANGING YOUR DIET. I HAVEN'T EVEN ADDED EXERCISE YET!**

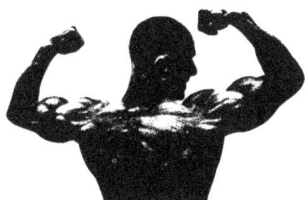

9

Shopping Like a Caveman Without the Club

Correct shopping is critical to a healthy lifestyle. Pretend you are a caveman in the grocery store. The only foods he would recognize would be fruits, vegetables, whole grains, nuts and eggs, right?

When I go shopping, I try not to walk the aisles; I stay on the perimeter. That is where the healthy, wholesome foods are located. First stop is for fruits and vegetables: sweet potatoes, broccoli, leafy greens, bananas, and asparagus. Next is the meat section for skinless, boneless chicken breasts, top sirloin, flank steak, 93 – 95% lean ground beef, pork tenderloin or fresh fish such as tilapia, sea trout or salmon. Finally, I pick up oatmeal (regular not instant), cinnamon and lots of eggs. If I use oil, it will be olive, grape seed, safflower seed or canola.

Helpful Hints:

Steam or roast broccoli or other vegetables ahead of time or just eat them raw after cleaning. Cook ahead a large number of chicken breasts, top sirloin, pork tenderloin or your selected lean meat and pack multiple small meals. If you have access to a microwave during the day, then carry uncooked sweet potatoes with you. If you do not have access to a microwave during the day, cook the potatoes in advance. Rice and pasta can also be prepared in advance. Place prepared food in storage containers or bags. This might sound tough, but give the idea a chance and you will see how simple it really is and everyday you will notice and feel the difference.

GROCERY CHECKLIST

DAIRY:
_____ Low fat cottage cheese
_____ Eggs

VEGETABLES:
_____ Asparagus
_____ Broccoli
_____ Snap peas
_____ Onions
_____ Lettuce
_____ Cucumbers
_____ Mushrooms
_____ Tomatoes
_____ Carrots
_____ Celery
_____ Sweet potatoes
_____ Cauliflower
_____ Potatoes
_____ Garlic
_____ Basil
_____ Parsley
_____ Cilantro
_____ Thyme

FRUITS:
_____ Bananas
_____ Strawberries
_____ Grapes
_____ Lemons
_____ Apples

SPICES:
_____ Pepper
_____ Dijon mustard
_____ Balsamic vinegar
_____ Worcestershire
_____ Cinnamon

MEAT:
_____ Skinless chicken breasts
_____ Ground beef (93%)
_____ Turkey breast
_____ Pork tenderloin
_____ Top sirloin
_____ Flank steak
_____ Buffalo

FISH:
_____ Tuna
_____ Tilapia
_____ Salmon

CANNED:
_____ Tuna, in water, low salt
_____ Salmon
_____ Tomatoes (no salt)
_____ Chick peas (garbanzo)
_____ Beans (black,lima, kidney)
_____ Olives

OTHER:
_____ whole-grain pasta
_____ Oatmeal
_____ Flax seed oil
_____ Sunflower oil
_____ Tea
_____ Almonds, no salt
_____ Sunflower seeds
_____ Brown rice
_____ Cashew butter
_____ Almond butter

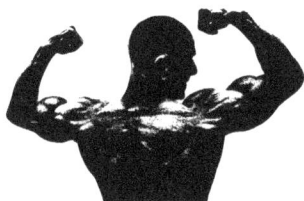

10

This is Simple, but I Cannot Cook!

You do not have to be a gourmet chef. You can cook while relaxing with your family, watching television or working on your computer. I plan, shop and prepare all my own foods ahead of time. I invite my young children to help me prepare meals so they learn about healthy habits while also spending time together. The more I teach people about how to do this, the more I am convinced that anyone who is motivated can follow the program. If you say you can do it, you will and your health will improve. Planning ahead and learning to prepare basic meals is your ticket out of an overweight world.

If you fail to plan then you plan to fail.

Let me help you break it down:

- To steam your favorite vegetable, place it in a steamer with a small amount of water and steam to desired level of doneness. For broccoli, peel the stem of the plant, cut into thin lengthwise strips and place in steamer with a small amount of water. Cover and steam on high for 12 minutes.

- To cook sweet potatoes, poke a hole in the potato and microwave on high for 5 to 6 minutes or bake in oven for one hour at 350 degrees.

- To cook chicken breast, top sirloin or 93% ground beef (as a hamburger patty), heat a nonstick pan on high, place meat in pan and cover for 3 minutes, turn and cover for 3 more minutes. Remove from heat, keep covered for 2 minutes and either serve, or place in a container for use at a later time. I usually cook multiple servings at once, that way I don't have to worry about not being prepared.

- Carry 4 containers with you for your 8 hour day. If you are traveling, place in a cooler along with your cold water.

Other variations of a meal could be a salad covered with four to six ounces of your desired meat with balsamic vinegar as dressing. I buy pre-cut salad, add slices of my favorite vegetables like cucumbers, onions, tomatoes, peppers, beans, mushrooms or black olives. I carry balsamic vinegar in a small container so I can add it when needed or use fat-free salad dressings.

I always carry a cooler with several of my prepared meals plus an extra one, just in case. Each plastic container contains meat, vegetables and potatoes. I also carry a plastic bag with one to two servings of my protein shake, water and a shaker so I can make a shake that tastes great and is full of healthy calories. Small frequent meals fuel my muscles and allow me to burn fat. Convenience store snacks such as chips, candy and sodas are unhealthy, full of chemicals and poisons that increase stored fat. Protein shakes do not cause a spike in insulin like processed snacks. Spikes in insulin on a continual basis can lead to diabetes.

Remember, preparation is key. The more you plan in advance, the less likely you are to have problems and the greater chance you have of being successful. Planning is crucial to your success. Modern day man has too many unhealthy choices and your preparation to carry wholesome food places you in the driver's seat.

What happens if I can't take my food with me or I am going to a restaurant?

When you are at a restaurant, ask for what you want and do not limit yourself to the menu. I frequently ask the server to prepare a salad with my meat of choice, grilled and placed on top. I ask for balsamic vinegar on the side. I have yet to find a restaurant unwilling to accommodate me. I ask for vegetables steamed with no butter or a sweet potato on the side. I rarely hear, "We can't do that." Also, ask what they put on your food when they grill it so you can be sure the meat is not covered in unhealthy fats. People go to restaurants to socialize and meet friends. You can still do this and eat the way you desire. Your family and friends will notice and maybe you can help other people with their eating habits. It is great to lead by example.

Remember, you may not be able to stick to these food choices ALL the time, but if you can follow the plan 50-75% of the time and make relatively healthy, educated choices the rest of the time, you will make huge changes within your one year goal. These are not novel ideas, just a new approach to the challenges of eating in an "on the go life." If you plan ahead and have healthy food nearby, you will not fail.

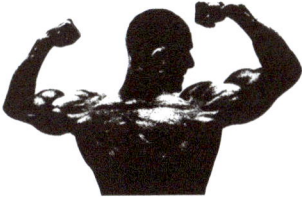

11

Eat Your Way to Success

> **Protein** is the major building blocks for muscles and most cells in your body.
>
> Think of protein as the bricks of a house.

Chicken breasts: Boneless, skinless chicken breast, bagged chicken breast tenderloin or ground white chicken breasts are great lean meat choices. Rotisserie whole chickens (breast meat only, skin removed) can also be found in most grocery stores. This is a convenient and easy way to get your protein without having to cook it yourself. Grilling chicken is another option. Grill plenty and use leftovers for future meals. Remember not to blacken the meats when grilling as some evidence points to this as a potential cancer source. (Jacobson, 2009)

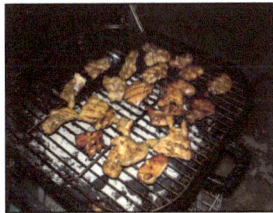

Fish: Fresh or frozen tuna, salmon, cod, tilapia or snapper are good fish choices as well. To prepare, bake or saute the fish in a small amount of olive oil. Do not fry. Vacuum-sealed packages of salmon or tuna are great alternatives. Canned white tuna in water is also convenient but avoid tuna in oils and buy ones with the lowest amount of sodium. A trick for flavor is to mix the tuna with mustard and spices of your choice. Limit your canned tuna intake to one can per day due to possible mercury contents.

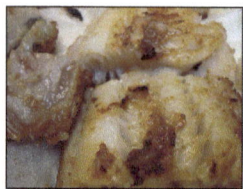

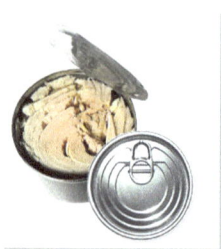

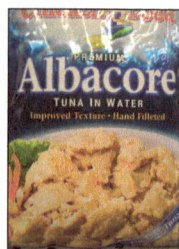

Turkey: Ground turkey breast 90% lean or leaner is a nice choice. Also, you can buy turkey breasts or turkey tenderloin. Roast turkey works well too, but concentrate on the white meat and no skin. No turkey legs, please.

Beef: Ground beef 93% or leaner, filet, top sirloin, top or bottom round and flank steaks are the leanest cuts of beef. Avoid fatty cuts of beef and read the labels for fat content. Buffalo is another healthy alternative.

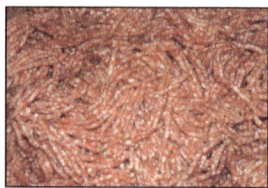

Pork: Pork tenderloin is an excellent source of lean protein and is easy to prepare. Ounce for ounce, pork tenderloin contains less fat than chicken breast. Also, fresh cuts do not contain nitrates or sodium, which may cause cancer or elevate your blood pressure. (Diet and Disease, 2009)

Deli meat: I do not recommend this, but if you are in a pinch, you can add some deli meat to your salad. Be sure to choose lean cuts and low sodium.

Egg whites: Eggs are an ideal source of protein. The average egg white from a large egg has 4-5 grams of protein. By separating out the yolk, you will avoid the cholesterol and fat. Egg substitutes contain larger amounts of sodium than pure egg whites.

Vegetables: Non-starchy vegetables are great for filling you up, so eat as much as you like. They are great sources of vitamins and minerals. Think of these as the cement that holds the bricks in place. Benefits from healthy fiber are well documented, including prevention of strokes, diabetes and cardiovascular disease. Vegetables also help decrease the absorption of cholesterol and unwanted fats. (Diet and Disease, 2009) Some suggestions include broccoli, asparagus, green beans, lettuce (all varieties), spinach, cauliflower, celery, cucumbers, onions, peppers (all varieties), squash (summer varieties only), eggplant and tomatoes.

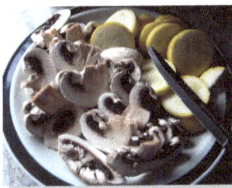

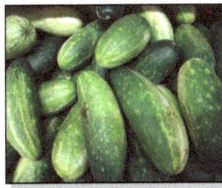

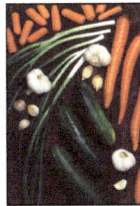

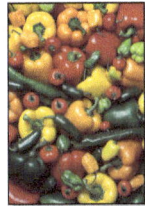

Carbohydrates: Starchy carbohydrates provide healthy fuel for your body if you chose the correct ones. They are also excellent sources of fiber. I recommend brown rice, sweet potatoes, red potatoes, Yukon potatoes, oatmeal, Cream of Rice, beans (black, lima, kidney and garbanzo), whole-grain pasta, and other grains such as millet and barley. Carbohydrates are the most abused and adulterated food group and responsible largely for the obese epidemic in America. Read the labels you are buying. If you see large amounts of simple sugars like fructose or sucrose, then do not buy the product. My suggestions are the complex carbohydrates that are good for you, especially when combined with lean meat and plenty of vegetables and fruits. Making poor choices with food items that contain simple carbohydrates (soda, fruit juices with high fructose corn syrup, chips, french fries, processed cereals) leads to obesity. Making correct choices is the key to weight loss and your continued success.

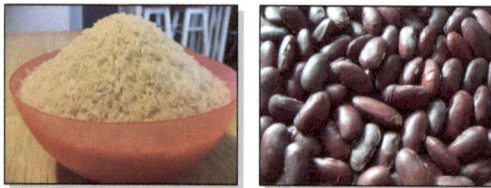

Fats: Fats are needed and there are some healthy types. Try cashew butter, almond butter, flaxseed oil, olive oil and sunflower oil. These food suggestions should be used as snacks or flavorings. These provide you with essential fats that actually assist with weight loss.

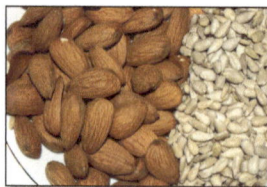

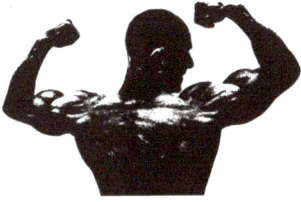

12

Foods You Must Avoid

We have all seen how cigarettes cause the lungs to be destroyed over time. Think of bad foods as destroying your body over time. Bad foods cause sludge to build up inside you just like sludge that builds up in your car if you do not change the oil. Treat yourself as well or better than you treat your car. Use the correct fuels and limit the foods that cause problems. Improperly fueling your body leads to weight gain, high blood pressure, heart disease and blocked arteries, which prevent blood from getting into your brain, heart, kidneys and legs.

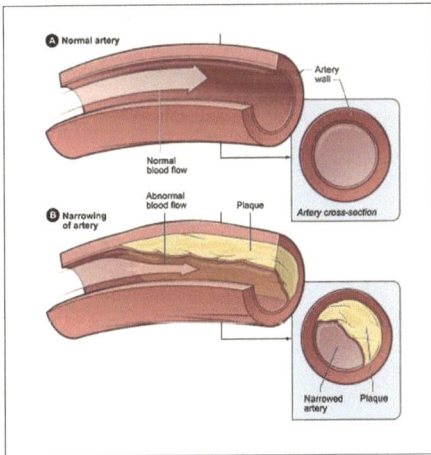

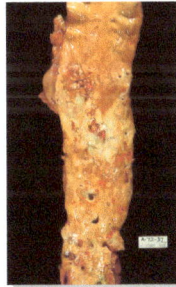

Above on the left is a comparison of a healthy artery with no disease and an artery with plaque. On the right is an unhealthy artery full of disease.

Stay away from the following types of foods

- Highly-processed foods
- Foods containing high fructose corn syrup, bleaches, flour, excess salt, fried foods, fruit juices, creamers, margarine, mayonnaise, munchies, chips, sugar, and processed wheat breads.

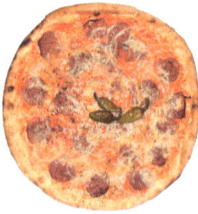

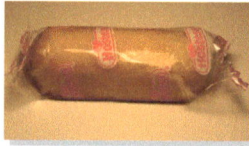

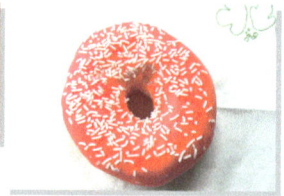

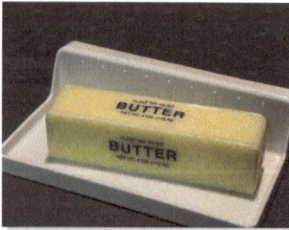

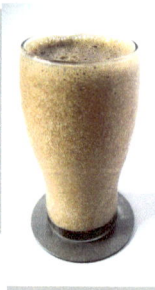

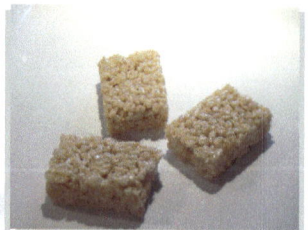

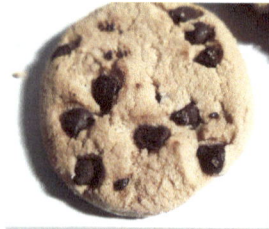

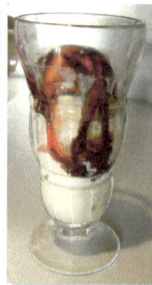

When it comes to breads, it is important to avoid even the "healthy" wheat and multi-grain varieties. These bread types are loaded with processed ingredients. Homemade freshly baked breads are acceptable, but you must limit yourself to very small amounts. If you are trying to lose weight, I suggest you avoid bread completely as it is very tempting to over eat and bread contains simple sugars that the body converts to fat.

When you are shopping, it is vital that you read the labels of food you intend to buy. If you see a long list of items, put it down and move on. This extensive list usually indicates the food item is highly-processed. Remember, if you cannot pronounce the ingredients, don't eat it.

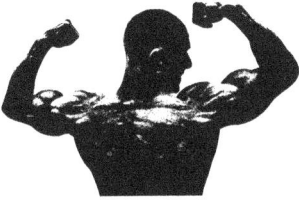

13

Supplements and Exercise

I take supplements for specific reasons: to help me work out longer, stronger and avoid soreness the next day. I also want to make sure I have the right vitamins and minerals in my body at all times. Supplements help me before and after I work out, help me sleep and feel better. They help mobilize fat from the storage deposits to the rest of the body for energy usage.

Supplements are not the complete answer. Eating healthy food is the answer. Think of supplements as an insurance policy that provides your body with the necessary nutrients for maximum performance.

I love working out. It always inspires me and gets my day off to a great start. I do more exercising before seven in the morning than most people do in a week. I am not bragging, but telling you this because this is who I have become over years of applying myself. Exercising clears my head and gets me thinking, which is how I came up with most of what you are reading.

Remember, caveman was always exercising. He had to hunt and work hard just to catch his food to survive and in doing so, he was constantly on the move. We are not so lucky. We have food available without doing hardly any work and as a result, we have gotten progressively lazier over time. This has resulted in a sedentary lifestyle which burns less fuel, consumes more calories and stores more fat.

Caveman was always walking or running, whereas modern-day man is using vehicles, elevators and escalators; all conveniences that lead to less energy being used. When at work, modern day man might sit at a computer using minimal physical energy and meanwhile, consuming unhealthy snacks leading to weight gain and complacency. This translates to health risks such as heart disease, diabetes and other preventable medical conditions. Small changes add up to big gains – in weight and physical fitness. If you do at least some activity, you burn more fuel. When you burn more fuel, you begin a process that leads to weight loss. I have explained the process; if you follow the plan, you will have a new and healthy approach to food which will help you lose weight and reach your ideal body weight in a healthy way.   Remember, quick fix weight loss prescription drug programs are full of side effects and carry inherent health risks. Consuming healthy foods does not have any side effects, except a healthier YOU.

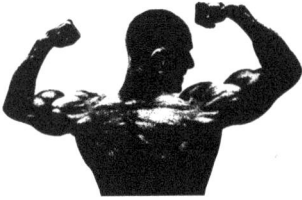

14

Pulling It All Together

> **"If you let life get in the way of your health, your health will get in the way of your life"**™
>
> -Mark N. Hashim, MD

I believe the above statement says it all. This summarizes why eating healthy and exercising is so vital to your body. Remember: it is YOUR body and only you can control what you do to your body and what you place in your body. This book discusses what you place in your body, concentrating on the correct fuel for your engine. By now, you understand putting unhealthy items in your body is like the wrong fuel in your gas tank.

I used to be _____.

I constantly hear people talk of their past glory days instead of how they made today a glorious day. Remember when you were a child, full of energy and able to run all day? You were probably a lot thinner, felt better, slept better and never got sore or aching muscles. Why are you now fatter, more tired, unable to sleep and sore after the slightest bit of exercise or movement?

The answer is simple – years of inactivity. I cannot be more direct. You and I both know it. Admit it and together, we can begin to overcome this problem. Together we will take small steps on a daily basis to make gains on a monthly and yearly basis. I have the utmost confidence that my simple program works and makes sense. I know this because I am living proof that a 47-year-old man can compete with persons half his age. How did I become this way? I made small gains every day, added a little more each month and before I knew it, I had become the mental image that I desired.

In other words, think of what you want to be and want to feel like. By making the right choices, **you will become that person**. You will be full of energy, able to play with your children and grandchildren, feel better, sleep better and know that you did so by eating healthy and exercising.

I am not asking you to go full throttle – we all know that if you push the limits too fast and too hard, you will break like a racecar. If you start off easy and add layers as you progress, you will become a lean, mean fighting machine – just like that rebuilt 1969 mustang. It takes time to progress from a piece of rusty, useless junk to a classic. You have to develop a plan, implement the plan and after a while, this action turns into a result. The same goes for your body. First, recognize that you have a problem. Then, figure out a plan (which I have now provided to you), start the plan, stick to the plan and before you know it, the results will occur. It is that simple. So let's begin to fix this broken machine. It was designed to be repaired and I will help you.

Following is a list that will help you with your weight loss goals and your *Healthy For Life Now* goals. Read it out loud, carry a copy with you, read them when you become frustrated or feel you are losing perspective. By doing so, you will stay focused. If you set your mind to it, your body will follow.

Simple Rules to Follow

- Write your goals on a mirror with a magic marker. Do not erase - this is your motivation staring at you every day. This helps you to be accountable to yourself. Now you're finally doing something for yourself that is positive and healthy.

- Eat and drink like a caveman. Caveman did not have processed foods, fruit juices, and sodas. Caveman did have access to water, meats, beans, oats, fruits and vegetables. Think about this, it makes sense.

- Limit all processed carbohydrates like bread, chips, crackers, items with ingredients you can't even understand (most items that are on the aisles of a grocery store). Eat large portions of vegetables. For flavoring use spices, balsamic vinegar or fat free dressings; avoid butter and margarine.

- Drink one ounce of water per pound of LEAN body weight per day. Therefore if you weigh 200 pounds, and have 25% body fat, drink 150 ounces of water.

- Always carry an emergency meal with you, such as chicken, broccoli and sweet potato; basically your favorite lean meat, complex carbohydrate and vegetable or fruit. You can also have a protein shake available. If you forgot to bring your meal, know places you can go to eat as healthful as possible.

- Take your ideal body weight, multiply by ten, and this is your caloric requirements for the day.

- Keep a log book of your daily weights and food intake. This makes you accountable.

- Eat a variety of foods as I have outlined to provide adequate amounts of the proper nutrition, which means the right carbohydrates, protein, fats, vitamins and minerals.

Simple Rules to Follow

- Effective planning helps eliminate the chances of eating poorly or skipping meals during your busy day.

- It takes 20 minutes for your brain to recognize you are full, so eat slowly because if you eat too fast you will think and feel you need more food

- If you're stuck and have to eat fast food, try Taco Bell® and order fresco style where they have removed most of the fat. Or try grilled chicken on a salad, and choose a light or fat free dressing; avoid the croutons and chips.

- Price per pound, eating my healthy diet is cheaper than eating unhealthy foods. The energy used by your body from these foods is far more efficient than that from unhealthy foods.

- Eating fattening foods makes you fat; eating lean foods makes you look lean.

- Weight gain occurs from lack of exercise and eating the wrong foods. Correct these two problems and weight loss will occur.

- Be realistic and anticipate setbacks and learn how to cope with them. List common problems and obstacles you might encounter and figure out in advance what you do when they occur.

- Tell everyone you know what you are trying to do. This helps you believe you can and your friends become your cheerleaders.

- Develop a sound and realistic plan to follow.

After 21 days of following this program, it now becomes a habit and soon it will be a lifestyle change. If you have stuck to this, you should be proud of yourself.

Don't say you can't do it, or else you will always fail. Say you can do it, and you will succeed.

Testimonials

I have known Mark Hashim personally for 26 years when we first met during our medical training. One thing has remained constant in those 26 years, and that is when Mark does anything and sets his goal, he does it to his absolute best which translates into him being the best at whatever he does. His energy and enthusiasm is unparalleled, and his refusal to accept "No" for an answer is his trademark. One of my friends jokingly describes him as "A pit bull in a shirt!" I seriously describe Mark as a person who is dedicated to constant and never ending improvement in all of his life's endeavors, and the person who has influenced my thinking to the point that my first reaction to new challenges is no longer, "I'm not sure I can do that" to an ingrained, "Yes, I can."

Once you combine Mark's discipline, energy, enthusiasm, goal-setting mastery, and positive mental attitude it becomes easy to understand why he is the best person to go to for advice, but when you add in his medical training, his M.D. degree, and his thorough understanding of human physiology from his training as an Anesthesiologist, it becomes a complete no-brainer that he is the best person to go to for all your training advice.

As a 48 year old out of shape Physician, I approached Mark with questions of what to do to achieve my fitness goals. He outlined an extremely simple diet plan, "Eat like a caveman," which simply means eating all natural whole foods with no processed foods. This consists of lean meats such as chicken breast, turkey breast, and lean hamburger as well as fish, egg whites, fat free cottage cheese, fibrous vegetables such as green leafy vegetables, oatmeal, sweet potatoes and various fruits. I followed his advice to eat 6 meals a day three hours apart. The meals are delicious, healthy, and I have not had a single hunger sensation or craving for other food since I made this permanent lifestyle diet change.

Continuing to follow Mark's advice, I began to exercise every day. I do 20 minutes on a recumbent bike while watching the morning news, or ESPN sports competition news. This is followed by 40 minutes of resistance weight training of various exercises on a 4 day split doing 5 sets of 12 for upper body and 5 sets of 15 for lower body.

I subsequently have dropped in weight from 188 pounds to 170 pounds in six weeks. I get compliments multiple times a day, and am in better shape and have a more muscular physique than my several nephews that are in their early twenties. I have tremendous energy during the day, I am never hungry, and I sleep like a stress-free rock! My goal is to drop another 10 pounds to arrive at my high school weight of 160, and this final stage is no longer a matter of "if", it is now a matter of "when", because as I've learned from Mark, "Yes, I can."

That's it. Eat like a caveman. Exercise every day, at least 20 minutes of aerobic cardiovascular work, and at least 40 minutes of resistance weight training. Follow Mark's educated and knowledgeable program which combines his Physician knowledge with his positive mental attitude. Mark told me the only thing stopping me from achieving my goals was me and he told me I no longer had any excuse. Now, you don't either! Look up, get up, and keep going!!!

Tom Lacey, M.D.

I was at the point of my life where I was so miserable and just did not care about my health.   I am 44 years old and went to see Doctor Hashim for a pain issue in my neck.   As I continued through my treatments I had asked him about a "Healthy" way to get back to the shape I felt when I was twenty.   Doctor Hashim suggested a workout routine as well as a diet plan, and then gradually expanded it as I felt better.   He promised me that if I would dedicate myself to his plan for just thirty days, I would feel and see a difference.   Thanks to Doctor Hashim's advice and support I have lost 11 lbs in 30 days going from 184 to 173 lbs and am back to running 5 miles a day.   My cardio has increased as well as my weight training and I am starting to see those six pack abs reappearing.   My quality of life is great; I enjoy outdoor activities and staying active.   I am truly starting to feel like I am twenty again.

Thanks Doctor Hashim
-Jon Macdonald

O ver the past year, Dr. Mark Hashim has been a great friend and coach in my efforts to take control of my physical conditioning.   I am closing in on 50 years of age, and over the last few years I have slowly but surely let myself go.   Since Mark has shared with me his approach of proper nutrition and exercise, I have lost over 25 pounds and I feel great again!   I realize that this is just the beginning, and that good health is not a "quick fix", but is a lifestyle.   I am committed to being healthy and with Mark's expertise and coaching, I know I will succeed.

Bob Lane

H ello, I wanted to take some time to thank you for taking such great care of me over the years. You are an awesome Doctor who I trust and am pleased with the comfort and compassion you have shared with me.   Again thank you for all that you do.

Sincerely,
Melissa Hanson

*L*et me start out by saying that I have had weight problems since I was a teenager. In my late forties to mid 50's I made it up to 310 pounds. That was a lot of weight to carry around. One Sunday afternoon I was so disgusted with myself because none of my work clothes fit so my wife and I went to the store to look for what I called my "fat clothes." My waist had expanded to a size 50, about the size of a 55 gallon drum and that's what I felt like. Needless to say, carrying all that weight around took its toll on my back. I have a new granddaughter now and I was having a problem even picking her up and keeping up with her. Most important, I felt I wasn't the same man my wife married 25 years ago.

Fast forward a few years and I went to be treated for my back pain by Dr. Mark Hashim. I was 296 pounds at that point and he told me more than once that l needed to lose weight to take the stress off my back. I suppose I could have opted to have my stomach stapled or taken diet pills but I didn't want to take that route. Dr. Hashim is such a health enthusiast and the more I talked to him about how he stays fit, the more interested I became. I had a talk with him one day about the young guys with the six pack abs and he raised his shirt and revealed that he is 47 years old and has a six pack.　I must say I was very impressed but you don't get to where he was by eating donuts and not exercising. This one conversation with the Doc started me on a path of weight loss. He told me about the things that he eats and does not eat. He gave me great suggestions for breakfast, lunch and dinner and even what to snack on. He explained about certain vitamins and natural supplements that I could add to my daily regimen of vitamins which could assist me in losing weight and getting my energy back.　I needed to change my life so, with the encouragement of my wife, I got started.

Trust me when I tell you I am just a regular guy that had to work for a living and pay his bills. I am just like you and felt the same way you do right now. You want to be able to look in the mirror and see a trim, healthy body that looks good in the clothes you're wearing. You want to have the energy to do the things you used to do. Because I listened to what Dr. Hashim explained to me about the body and the fuel you put into it, I can now say that I am 58 years old and have never felt better about myself. Yes, it took me ten months and some *willpower and resolve to get down to my current weight of 245 pounds, but that is down 65 pounds from the day I went to buy the "fat clothes", and I am not finished yet! With the encouragement from Dr. Hashim and my family, I plan to lose another 25 pounds and maybe more. I could not believe that my waist size was down to a 38, which is what it was when I was in high school. This was accomplished with very minimal exercise although I would like to start working on firming up my new body in addition to trimming a few more pounds.*

I am thankful each day that I had a professional like Dr. Hashim, who took an interest in sharing his knowledge with a patient and guiding me on the right path to a better me.

Frank McDowell, III

BEFORE

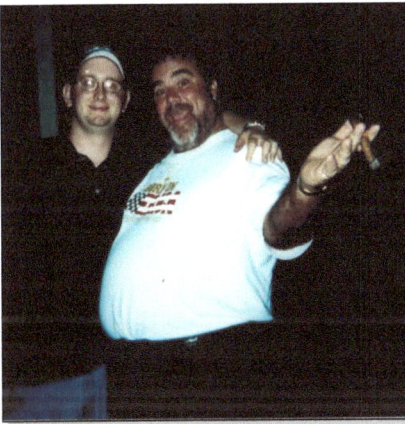
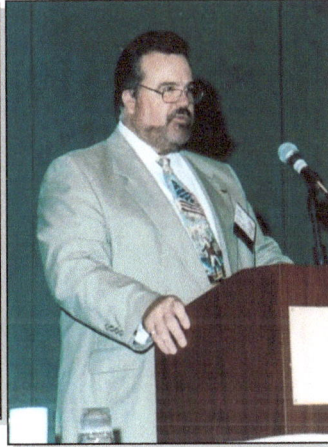

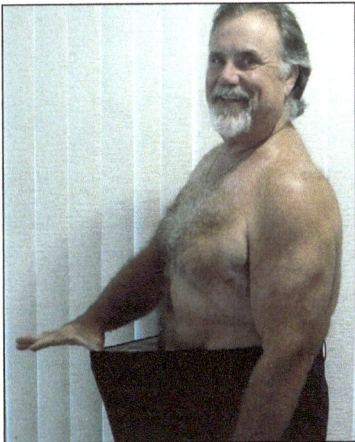

AFTER

*E*very once in a long while, I come across someone who truly puts another person's welfare ahead of their own pocketbook. You, my friend, definitely have fallen into that category. Having been one of your chronic pain patients for many years, I must admit that I carried a few too many pounds on my 5'9" frame, two hundred and fifty five as of the last week in January. That's according to my scale, not yours.

I know that you tried for many years to nudge me into doing something about my 'little weight problem' but I just wasn't ready for the hassle of going on another diet. Too much work for too little reward. After returning from another gluttonous cruise in January, you looked at me and finally had enough of my ignoring your gentle suggestions. This time you simply laid down the law regarding my future. Do something about my lifestyle or die at an early age. This really hit home. Now was the time to step up and do something. I just didn't know what 'something' was.

The time you spent with me providing suggested lifestyle changes rather than another diet really hit home. Not only were they relatively easy to follow, but they worked. Now twelve weeks later, I've already lost 49 pounds without missing a meal or ever feeling hungry. Taking ninety percent of your advice with ten percent of my tweaking to accommodate my personal tastes, allowed me to buy into the philosophy. I'm well on my way to the 'new, lighter' me.

Your slightly more than gentle prodding got me on the right track even though it has cost you some money. So far, I've been able to reduce the number of procedures you perform each month by half. Sorry for your loss of funds, but again thanks for putting me and my well-being ahead of your wallet. You have truly shown just where your degree of caring and lifestyle philosophy for your patients fits into your personal priorities.

Forever grateful,
Gary Blumberg

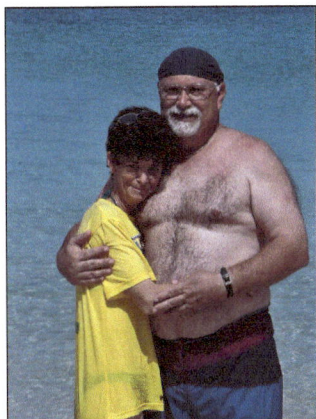

BEFORE

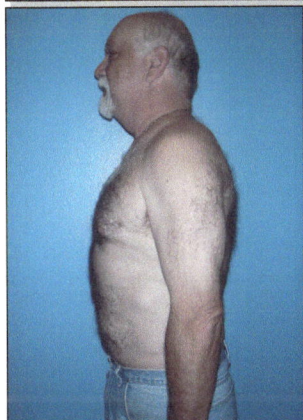

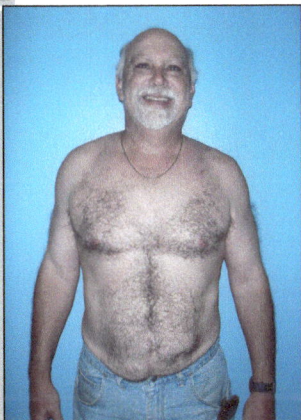

AFTER

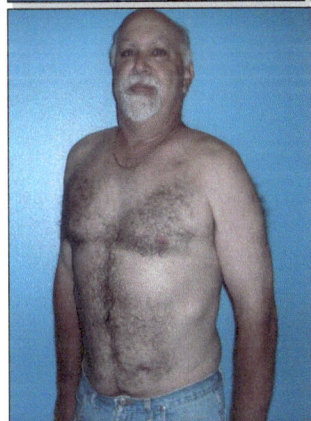

*M*y name is Chad and I am a patient of Dr. Mark Hashim. I have been diagnosed with spondylolisthesis, degenerative disc disease, and sciatica. I am limited to certain activities but that has not stopped me, with Dr. Hashim's help, in improving my health. I see Dr. Hashim for treatment and during my time with him, he has introduced me to a number of health products that have changed my way of living, not a diet, a change in "Life Style." With his help, by following his program, I have lost 63 pounds. I feel like a new person! THANK YOU DR. HASHIM!!!

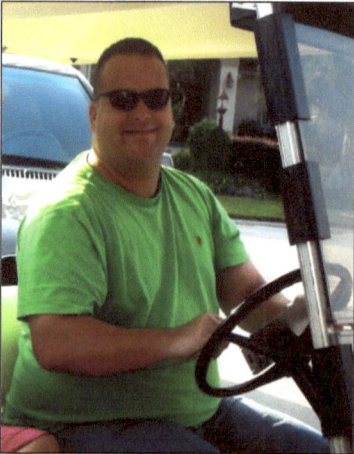

BEFORE

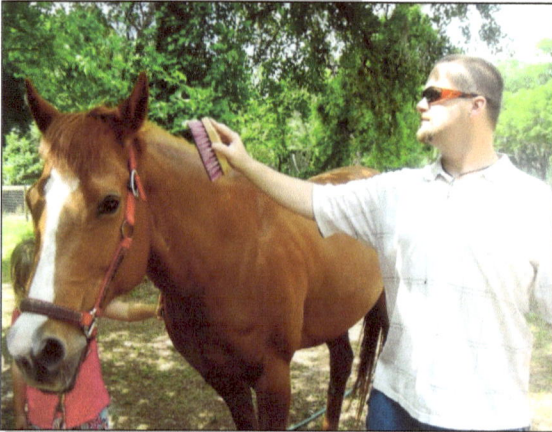

AFTER

Dear Dr. Hashim,

I would like to thank you for everything you have done for my husband. As you know, when Tim started coming to you for pain control, due to multiple back surgeries, his right leg was considerably atrophied and he required a cane for ambulation. Now, thanks to your ability to motivate as well as your vast knowledge of diet and exercise, he's no longer dependent on the cane 100% because his leg strength has greatly improved and muscle mass increased.

It is very difficult for anyone with limited mobility to lose weight, but since you customized a diet and exercise regime to meet Tim's specific needs he has been able to lose 27 pounds thus far.

You have an incredible gift to motivate people to better themselves. Tim always leaves your office encouraged to do better. Once again thank you for improving Tim's quality of life (and mine).

Sincerely,
Michele & Tim Thomasson

Thank you for telling it like it __IS__ in your book!! The book makes so much sense and is so easy to follow. There are lots of great helpful hints and best of all the weight is coming off and I am __not__ hungry!! Also the supplements you recommended are fantastic. Imagine energy without the jitters!!! I love it!!!

Thank you again,
Gayle

Thanks Doc! Wow, what a difference a couple years can make. When we first meet I was 250 pounds plus. My body was in bad shape. But here's the funny thing, I thought I was in pretty good shape. Yes I was heavy, my back hurt, I had high blood pressure and I smoked like crazy etc... At 45 I was just going thru life. I remember you asking me if I had any plans to change my life style. I said no I don't think so. I thought I was doing fine. As I'm getting ready to get a couple of shots in my lower back, you said something like well if you are not going to change at 45, then at the rate your going by the time your 55, if you make 55, you will weigh about 275 plus pounds and if you think you got problems now, just you wait and see what happens if you don't change. At first I was like damn I'm 45, I've got to change, so okay how do I do it? You recommended that I start slow. You told me you did not get here over night, you are not going to lose it over night. Try to lose one pound a week. I realized that I can do that. So I started your program and two years later I'm in the best shape of my life. I have lost over fifty five pounds and I feel great, and look great. And as you know, there are no more shots for me. If folks will try your program Doc, it will change their lives forever. I am living proof.

Thanks,
Paul Hloska

*M*y Name is Pamela Hammersley, and I lost my left leg to the hip in a motorcycle accident twenty-three years ago. I weighed 224 at the beginning of May and now at the end I've lost six pounds this month from making some small changes in my lifestyle that Dr. Hashim advised me to make. Those are to drink much more water and to wean off sodas, which is hard because I was addicted to soda. People talk about addiction to artificial sweeteners, sugar, caffeine and processed flours. I agree with the opinion that you need to wean off of these substances in order to ensure your success, otherwise you find yourself caving in to the cravings. Dr. Hashim's advice and good example of an embodiment of health, really helped motivate me to stick with it, to give my taste buds that time to change to where those things are no longer tasteful to them and to start up an exercise regime, starting off slowly and building up to longer work-outs and more repetitions as I could tolerate it. If I can do it you can too! You're not alone in going down the path of weight loss, and the journey of a thousand paces begins with just one. Just be persistent with envisioning your results and your results will come.*

I have suffered from arthritis for most of my adult life and have undergone 11 operations and have 6 artificial joints. In 2009 I went to see Dr. Mark Hashim for pain management. He gave me some epidural injections in my spine and some trigger point injections in my trapezius muscle. For years I had trouble turning my head because of the severe pain in my traps. Dr. Hashim instructed me in the proper technique for doing shrugs and my traps have been pain free for over a year. I also asked him about medical weight loss and his response was that I was an educated person who should eat right and exercise. Well I stewed over that advice for a few weeks and on January 1st of 2010 I began exercising and haven't looked back. I have since lost 16 pounds and feel great. I am on no pain medications and when my back flares up Dr. Hashim treats me without drugs. He has truly changed my life and he is an inspiration to me.

Mike Imparato, Age 49

*M*y husband Ron and I are starting your "caveman diet" today. Wish we had done this 20 years ago but it is never too late. Thanks so much for your website and your talk about the way to live and eat. You look wonderful.

Sincerely,
Joyce A. Sheffler and Ron Sheffler

About the Author

I have always been involved in fitness from the time I was growing up in Rockville, Maryland. When I was 16, I completed my first marathon after a friend told me I couldn't do it. I really dislike the word "can't" and I enjoy proving people wrong about my physical capabilities. I was awarded with the Scholar Athlete of the Year in high school. I became extremely interested in weight training and found that it came naturally and was an excellent complement to the sports I competed in including soccer, cross country and track and field. I continued to train with weights while attending Swarthmore College and competing in cross country. I also completed two marathons and another ½ marathon one week after a full because someone told me I couldn't do it.

While in medical school, I continued to weight train and run on a daily basis. I completed one more marathon and then completed a triathlon after a friend told me I could not complete one while in medical school. I graduated from the University of Pittsburgh School of Medicine in 1989 with honors and continued to work out while completing an anesthesia residency at the Medical College of Virginia in Richmond. I decided after my residency to apply my weight training to power lifting and won the two competitions I entered in the 148 weight class. While preparing for this competition, my trainers introduced me to the VersaClimber by Heart Rate, Inc. I firmly believe this to be a cornerstone of any fitness program.

When I moved to Florida to enter private practice in anesthesia, I continued to weight train and bicycled 40-75 miles a day. When my second child was born, I purchased my VersaClimber. After several months, I was in top physical condition working out at a 20 year olds heart rate in a 43 year olds body. I continued to weight train using my power lifting routines and began to notice outstanding definition occur. I then began to perfect my nutrition and started to add supplements.

Everything was improving and then disaster struck. While on vacation, I went to the gym for my usual work out and left the gym feeling good. Three hours later, I developed a discomfort in my left side at the origin of my left long head of triceps. Ten minutes later my first, second and third fingers went numb. Being a Pain Management physician I knew something horrible had occurred. One half hour later, I developed sudden paralysis of my left long head triceps and left pectoralis major. These muscles were paralyzed! I could not do one push up and could not even bench 20 pounds with my left arm! I was totally unable to flex any of these muscles. An MRI showed a huge ruptured disc in my neck totally compressing the nerve. This cut off the blood supply to the nerve therefore the nerve died and was unable to send information to the affected muscles. Over the next two weeks my left triceps and pectoralis major completely atrophied. Thirty years of training gone in two weeks! I lost 4 inches in the circumference of my left arm and my pectoralis major (chest) disappeared. I consulted top neurosurgeon, Dr. Steven Bailey in Gainesville, Florida who informed me that we had to do emergency surgery or risk forever completely losing these muscle groups. I had an anterior cervical disc removal and a PEEK disc (synthetic) placed between the 6th and 7th vertebrae. I never took a pain pill and started my comeback the very next day in the gym. I was frustrated and got very depressed when I realized this was going to be a trying treacherous course. I could not even triceps extend 5 pounds or bench a 15 pound dumbbell with my left arm. My neighbor, a physician, told me before my surgery that I would never recover...never. Remember I can't stand being told I can't do something especially when it is physical. It took about 220 days from the time of my surgery and daily workouts for my nerve to finally regenerate and muscle contraction began to occur. I then set a goal to compete for the first time in bodybuilding and to win my class no matter what. This I achieved on March 27, 2010 at the Northern Kentucky NPC Bodybuilding Championships.

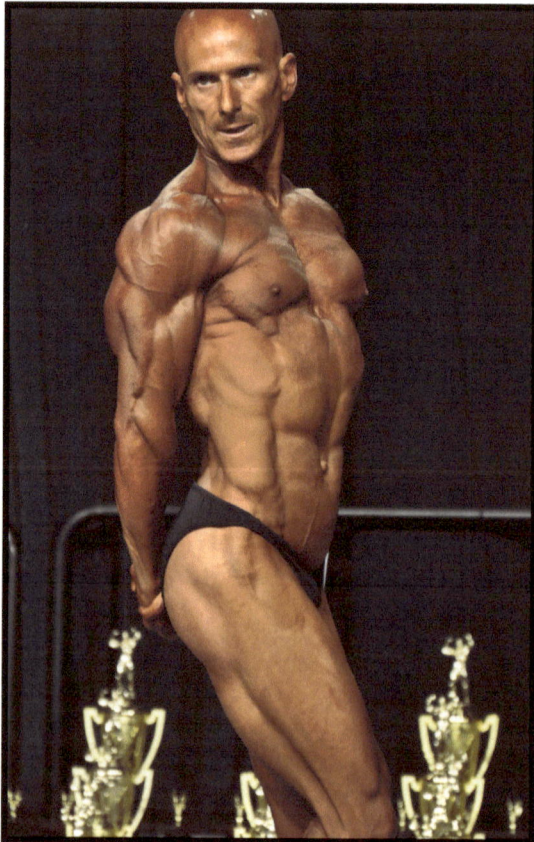

"Live your dreams, always do your best, don't ever give up, always believe you can, never ever believe you can't."

Mark N. Hashim, M.D.

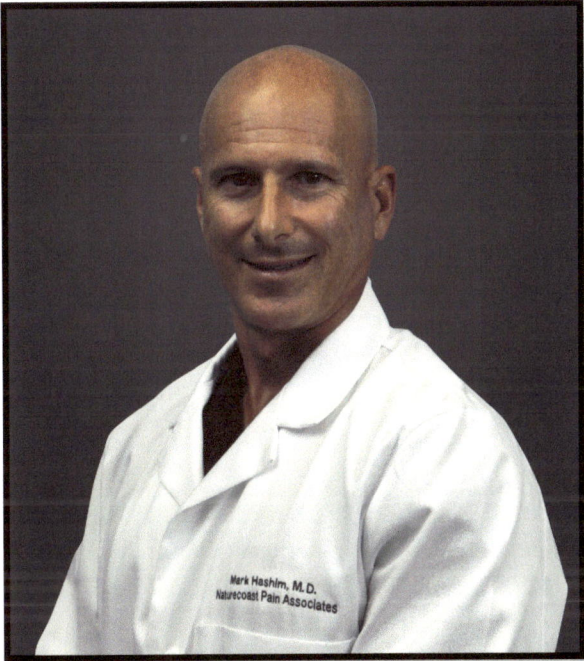

REFERENCES

American Heart Association. (2010). *Heart disease and stroke statistics – 2010 update.* Retrieved from http://www.american heart.org/presenter.jhtml?identifier=3018163.

Boschmann, M., Steiniger, J., Hille, U., Tank, J., Adams, F., Sharma, A., Klaus, S., Luft, F. (2003, Dec). Water induced thermogenesis. *Journal of Clinical Endocrinology and Metabolism*, 88(12), 6015-6019.

Brownell, Kelly. (2010, May). In your face. *Nutrition Action Healthletter,* 37(4), 3-6.

Dugdale, M.D., David. (Reviewed 2009). *Diet and disease.* Retrieved from http://adam.about.com/encyclopedia/Diet-and-disease.htm.

Fowler, S., Williams, K., Resendez, R., Hunt, K., Hazuda, H., Stern, M. (2008). Fueling the obesity epidemic? Artificial sweetened beverage use and long-term weight gain. *Obesity*, 16(8), 1894 - 1900.

Jacobson, Micheal. (2008, May). Chemical cuisine. *Nutrition Action Healthletter,* 35(4), 3-8.

Jacobson, Michael. (2009, June). The real cost of red meat. *Nutrition Action Healthletter,* 36(5), 3-7.

1. My overall goal is to lose _____ pounds.

2. My goal will take me _____ weeks. (assume 1 pound per week)

3. I will reach my goal by _____. (enter date)

4. Write on your mirror your goal and your target date.

5. Calculate your <u>ideal</u> body weight then multiply by 10.

     _____ x 10 = _____ total calories per day

     Then divide by 6 = _____ total calories per meal

AMOUNT OF PROTEIN, COMPLEX CARBOHYDRATE AND GOOD FATS PER MEAL: (ASSUMING 6 MEALS/DAY)

6. Calculate the number of total grams of protein per day. This is equal to your ideal body weight = _____

7. Calculate total grams of protein per meal by taking your total protein per day (as above) and divide by 6 (assuming 6 meals/day) _____

8. Calculate total grams of carbohydrates per meal. Take total calories per day and multiply by 0.01458 = _____

9. Calculate total fat grams per meal. Take total calories per day and multiply by 0.004629 = _____ .

10. I will eat 6 meals a day with _____ grams of protein,

     _____ grams of complex carbohydrates, and

     _____ grams of fats.

IF I FOLLOW THIS PLAN I WILL REACH MY GOAL WEIGHT OF _____ POUNDS BY _____ (enter date).

11. I will write down what I eat at each meal and what time I eat my meals. I will write down my protein, carbohydrate and fat eaten at each meal. I will write down how much water a day I drink and how many calories I consumed.

Example Meal	Time	Protein (grams)	Carbs (grams)	Fat (grams)	Water (oz)
1	07:00	6 Egg Whites 26	½ cup Oatmeal 27	1 ½ tsp Olive Oil 7	Water 20
2	09:30	3 oz Chix Breast 25	½ cup Brown Rice 22	1 ½ tsp Olive Oil 7	Water 20
3	12:00	4 oz Lean Burger 26	½ cup Sweet Potato 20	From Burger 7	Water 20
4	14:30	3 oz Tuna 25	½ cup Sweet Potato 20	1 ½ tsp Olive Oil 7	Water 20
5	17:00	6 Egg Whites 26	½ cup Oatmeal 27	1 ½ tsp Olive Oil 7	Water 20
6	19:30	3 oz Top Sirloin 26	½ cup Sweet Potato 20	From Steak 7	Water 20
Total		154 GRAMS	132 GRAMS	42 GRAMS	120 oz
		616 Calories	528 Calories	378 Calories	1422 Total Calories

(Hint: To use a simple food calculator, I recommend www.nutritiondata.com)

12. I will weigh myself every week and write down my progress.

TO IMPROVE MY WEIGHT LOSS, I WILL BEGIN TO SLOWLY ADD EXERCISE TO MY PROGRAM

13. To start exercising I will begin by walking for 10 minutes my first day and add 1 minute every day until I can walk for 20 minutes.

14. I will continue to exercise every day trying to walk faster and further during my 20 minutes.

15. After 2 months, I will begin to add 1 minute per day until I am walking for 30 minutes every day.

www.ingramcontent.com/pod-product-compliance
Lightning Source LLC
Chambersburg PA
CBHW041217270326
41931CB00001B/6